Using Aromatherapy Diffusers:

Selecting Essential Oils, Creating Blends and Choosing a Diffuser

Joy Bennett

©2015 Dilettante Living Press

Publisher: Dilettante Living Press

Cover Design: Vikiana

Contents

Chapter 1: Why aromatherapy?

People have been harnessing the power of plants to cure their ailments for centuries. Evidence of the use of essential oils can be found as early as in Egyptian times, but may have existed in China even before then. With the advent of modern medicine the popularity of herbal remedies waned, but aromatherapy has enjoyed a resurgence in popularity in recent decades as people are turning away from synthetics and back toward nature. And, while our forefathers relied on ancient wisdom and some trial and error when healing with plant oils, we now have scientific evidence that essential oils do provide health benefits. What is aromatherapy? The definition lies in the word itself—using *aroma*tic compounds for *therap*eutic results. Or, in simpler terms, using plant oils to help the body achieve and maintain health. Health includes both physical and emotional wellness. Aromatherapy can be used to:

°Assist in maintaining physical health

°Ease emotional concerns

°Scent your environment without chemicals

You can even achieve all three of these at once, depending on which oils you choose to use. This book will show you how aromatherapy works by diffusion (inhalation) as an alternative or supplement to aromatherapy massage. Once we have covered the basics we will look at some of the specific essential oils and their uses in a diffuser, as well as discuss factors to consider when choosing aromatherapy diffusers. By the end of this book, I hope that you will be armed with all you need to know to diffuse essential oils in your home safely and effectively.

Why use diffusers?

Essential oils can be used in two main ways—by applying them topically (well diluted) or by inhaling them. You may see some sources suggest that you can also ingest them however most major aromatherapy associations do not recommend this unless under the personal guidance of a qualified expert. While either method of administration can be used, topical administration may be particularly well suited for skin issues, water retention, relaxation, pain, and gastrointestinal issues. Inhalation may be more useful for respiratory complaints, stress and anxiety, immune stimulation and disinfection.

When essential oils are applied topically, they enter the body through the skin via absorption. It is crucial that you never apply essential oils to the skin neat. They must be diluted in a base such as a carrier oil (e.g. olive oil, sweet almond oil, etc.), a lotion, a balm or salve, etc. Typical dilutions are 1-2% essential oils to 98-99% base product. This may seem like very little but essential oils are very concentrated— in some cases it takes several hundred pounds of plant material to yield one ounce of essential oils. To illustrate just how concentrated they are, consider that it takes about 9 pounds of lavender to make one ounce of essential oil. Pouring one ounce of lavender oil in your bathtub is like bathing with 135 cups of lavender! To achieve the same effect as one cup of lavender buds in the tub, you only need about 5 drops of essential oil. Because of the concentrated nature of essential oils, some people may experience sensitivity reactions to certain oils when applied topically.

When essential oils are absorbed into the skin they make their way into the bloodstream. There is some debate, however, as to just how much essential oil makes it into the bloodstream. Martin Watt[1] makes the argument that when volatile essential oils contact warm skin, much of the oil will evaporate before it can penetrate into the skin. Despite this theory, research demonstrating the efficacy of topical administration (through aromatherapy massage) exists. However, these studies have the limitations of not being able to control for the effect of inhaling the aroma during massage, nor for the beneficial response to massage itself. Therefore we cannot be sure if the observed effects are because of absorption of essential oils into the skin or if some of the effects came from inhalation of the aroma or the healing touch of the massage.

By contrast, when essential oils are inhaled, researchers have found appreciable levels of essential oils in the bloodstream. When we diffuse essential oils into the air, we are benefiting from the emotional response to the scent (much as we respond to the scents of different perfumes or the smell of a campfire) as well as allowing essential oils to enter our lungs and bloodstream. Oils that enter our bodies through inhalation affect us in two ways. The aroma and molecules of the essential oil enters through the nose and registers with our olfactory system. The molecules are also inhaled into the lungs where they are transferred into our bloodstream and circulate throughout our bodies before being excreted. When you breathe in air with essential oils suspended in it, both processes occur simultaneously.

The olfactory system

Certain smells can carry us back to a place and time. The smell of apple pie might remind us of grandmother's house, or the smell of cloves may remind us of the dentist's office. Smells can trigger these emotions and memories before we are even able to consciously identify the scent. The emotions and memories that are brought to the surface may be pleasant, or not. That is why when choosing which essential oils to use it is not just about what oil can serve what purpose—you must find the scent pleasing if you are to enjoy using it.

When essential oil molecules enter your nose, they are caught by cilia in the lining of the upper nose. This causes receptors to send messages to the olfactory bulb, which lies between the roof of our nasal cavity and the brain. The olfactory bulb sends this information to the olfactory cortex of the brain as well as to the limbic system. The olfactory cortex is the area of the brain that processes scent information. More interesting however is the limbic system, which is associated with emotions, learning, hunger, sex drive, and hormonal functions. It is thought that different essential oil molecules trigger different hormones to be released. For example, some molecules may stimulate the release of serotonin, which has the effect of relieving anxiety. So, when we smell an odor, it not only triggers an emotional response, but a physiological one as well.

Inhalation into the lungs

When we diffuse essential oils in our home, essential oil molecules are dispersed into the air we breathe. The air that we inhale goes into our lungs all the way down into the small sac like endings called alveoli. This means inhalation can be a great way to treat some respiratory diseases due to direct contact of the oils with lung tissue. Alveoli are surrounded by capillaries. An exchange occurs where oxygen and other molecules are transferred into the bloodstream and waste products are transferred out. The blood transports inhaled molecules throughout the body. It is estimated that at rest it only takes one minute for blood to circulate through the entire body. Inhalation is therefore a quick and easy way to get essential oil molecules into our circulatory system.

The benefits of inhalation as a method of administering essential oils are then that it works simultaneously by stimulating the olfactory and limbic systems as well as efficiently transporting essential oil molecules throughout the body via the circulatory system. And it does this with much lower risks due to the dilution of essential oils into the entire volume of room air rather than a few ounces of a topical base. Furthermore, it can be safer as direct skin contact is avoided, thereby reducing the possibility of skin sensitivity reactions. We now know the benefits of inhalation as a way to experience essential oils, the next chapter examines how the oils themselves affect our health.

Chapter 2: Benefits of Aromatherapy

Diffusing essential oils can help us to achieve and maintain physical and emotional wellness as well as scent our environment naturally. This chapter examines these benefits in more detail. Essential oils can be used to help keep us healthy by:

°Stimulating the immune system (disease prevention)

°Antimicrobial activity (killing bacteria, viruses, and fungi)

°Complementary therapy for specific medical issues

Using aromatherapy for a healthy body

1. Stimulating the immune system

Some essential oils such as tea tree, lemon, and lavender are thought to strengthen the immune system. Exposure to these oils is said to stimulate production of white blood cells, which are an important component of our immune systems. Furthermore, lavender has a relaxing effect and is useful in times of stress. We know that we are more susceptible to getting sick when we are under stress, so reducing stress is certainly a factor in maintaining a healthy immune system. A stronger immune system means fewer illnesses and a body that is better equipped to quickly fight off disease when it does succumb.

2. Antimicrobial activity

All essential oils are antiseptic. Many essential oils have specific components that make them anti-bacterial, anti-viral, or anti-fungal. Some, like tea tree oil, are all three. Many common diseases are bacterial or viral in nature. Antibiotics can help cure bacterial infections, but there are fewer options for viruses. That is why your doctor tells you to go home and rest when you have a virus—you need to let your body fight the virus because aside from prescription antivirals, there is no medicine to combat viruses. This is where nature wins out over conventional medicine. Medicines and vaccines are difficult to formulate because viruses change and mutate so frequently. Essential oils are thought to not be affected by problems such as bacterial resistance and mutating viruses. So, it may be possible to reduce the duration and/or symptoms of a virus with essential oils.

One of the most famous examples of the power of essential oils to prevent disease is the story of grave robbers during the bubonic plague who managed to avoiding getting sick while dealing with the corpses and belongings of those who had succumbed to the plague. When they were caught, they were offered leniency if they agreed to divulge their secret. It turns out that they used plants and herbals to protect themselves. While the exact concoction varies in the telling, most modern blends based on the story of the thieves include Cinnamon, Clove, Lemon, Rosemary and Eucalyptus, all of which are powerful antiseptic oils.

History also gives us accounts of perfumers and glove makers in France during the 17th century who were reputed to rarely get sick. Both professions involved using essential oils on a daily basis (gloves were perfumed with essential oils). My own experience coincides with others-- since beginning to diffuse essential oils myself and my family have noticed fewer illnesses, illnesses that are milder, and we get better faster.

How does one use essential oils to accomplish this? Let's take a moment to examine how essential oils can work to combat illness through stimulating the immune system and through their antimicrobial activity. Disease needs two things to fall into place in order for a person to get sick:

°Exposure to the germ in an infectious dose

°A susceptible host

The first point, exposure to the bug in an infectious dose means that you need to come in contact with enough of the bug to get you sick. Now, this can be a very little amount, but it is also possible to come in contact with a sick person and not get sick yourself. Health care workers who have been accidentally stuck by a needle contaminated with HIV have not gotten the virus. Why? Because there wasn't enough of the virus on the needle to infect them. On the other hand, it is possible to get sick just from touching something that a sick person has touched, like a doorknob. Keeping surfaces clean and good hand washing habits are your first line of defense against everyday diseases. Essential oils can supplement this by disinfecting both surfaces in a room as well as the air. The second most important factor in reducing your risk of exposure to an infectious dose of a germ is to avoid touching places where bugs can get into your body, namely your mouth, nose, and eyes.

One research study demonstrated that when Geranium and Lemongrass were diffused in a room, it reduced airborne bacteria by as much as 89% (Doran, Morden, Dunn, Edwards-Jones, 2009)[2]. Another study in a hospital setting found a reduced incidence of MRSA when essential oils were diffused (BBC News)[3]. MRSA is a strain of staphylococcus aureus that is resistant to most antibiotics which makes this result even more impressive. Besides reducing airborne microbes, surfaces in a room where essential oils had been vaporized had a lower level of contamination by microbes (Doran, et al., 2009). These results suggest that diffusing essential oils can help to reduce both airborne and surface microbes in a room. Fewer airborne and surface microbes in a room means a decreased chance of coming into contact with an infectious dose.

The second factor needed to get ill is a susceptible host. A virus needs a host to occupy in order to reproduce and function. If the host's defenses are strong enough, it is possible to stop the virus before it has a chance to replicate to the point where you begin to experience the symptoms of being sick. When you take actions to strengthen your immunity such as eating a healthy diet, exercising, and using immunostimulant essential oils, you are increasing your body's ability to fight that infectious dose. Again, this can mean preventing disease from occurring, lessening symptoms, or shortening the duration of an illness.

3. Complementary therapy for medical conditions

Many essential oils have been identified as being particularly helpful for certain conditions. For example, oils such as eucalyptus or peppermint are often used to ease sinus issues. Peppermint and lavender can be helpful if you have a headache. Chapter 5 will discuss some of the oils that can be used for specific situations or you can consult with a clinical aromatherapist who can make individualized recommendations. Seeking expert advice is particularly important if you have a complex medical history. If you are in good health using this book, or one of several excellent books by experts in the field may be all you need.

Using aromatherapy for emotions and mood

Have you ever drawn a hot bath, lit some scented candles and felt the tensions of the day just melt away? If so, you have used scents to alter your mood. Just imagine now that you used pure essential oils to set this mood instead of synthetic candle scents? Just as you can address specific physical conditions with essential oils, you can also address emotional ailments. Essential oils can set a mood (such as romantic or calming at the end of a busy day) but they can also help with conditions such as stress, anxiety or depression.

Lavender is well known for having a calming effect and is one of the recommended oils for stress and relaxation. Other oils such as Bergamot can assist with anxiety. Sometimes we don't want to alleviate a complaint, but we want to enhance performance. Once again, there are essential oils for the job. Some oils are stimulating and can be used to heighten focus and concentration. These oils might be employed while driving a car or studying for a big test. Chapter 5 has more suggestions for specific uses of essential oils for emotional issues and mood enhancement.

Using aromatherapy to scent a home naturally without chemicals

More and more people are aware that the chemical burden on our body has gotten out of hand in the last century. We put more and more chemicals into our bodies, on our bodies, into the earth. Synthetic air fresheners are full of chemicals and manufacturers do this because man-made scents are cheaper and more consistent to produce than natural scents. Just as the climate and soil used to grow grapes can affect a wine's flavor from year to year, growing conditions for the plants that are used for essential oils vary from year to year. This can result in inconsistency of the scent of the essential oil from one year to the next. Synthetic scents smell exactly the same year after year so manufacturers opt for consistency.

Some air fresheners not only mask odors with their scent, but may actually interfere with your sense of smell by coating your nasal passages with an oily substance. Personally, I hate the way synthetic perfumes, body sprays and air freshener's smell. Their scent gets stuck in my nose and throat for hours. Interestingly, essential oils do not produce this effect and I actually enjoy their scent. I believe that is my body telling me something!

Essential oils are the inspiration for many synthetic scents, so in some cases you can re-create your favorite scents using natural essential oils. I discuss some tips for blending your own scents in Chapter 5. Of course it is important to remember when using essential oils for scents that some possess similar actions and precautions as medications so they must be used prudently. Chapter 3 talks more about safety, and we mustn't be led to believe that natural oils will necessarily be safer than man-made oils. You must choose wisely and educate yourself as to what essential oils are safe to use on a regular basis and more importantly, which are not.

Chapter 3: Before you start—important safety precautions

According to the National Association of Holistic Aromatherapists[4], inhalation is generally a safe method of using essential oils. This is because we are diluting the essential oil into the volume of air in the room. They state that even in a small closed room with 100% evaporation of an oil, a toxic concentration of oil is unlikely. They do add the caution however that prolonged use may lead to nausea, vertigo, headaches, or lethargy, so let's not go crazy with diffusing!

There is a general misconception that natural products are inherently safer than man-made chemicals. This is not always true. There are several plants that are deadly to humans. Other plants can cause liver damage if overused (e.g. Comfrey root). The FDA regulates drugs in the United States but it does not require herbal supplements, including essential oils, to prove their safety and efficacy before going on the market. Studies are being conducted on essential oils but as of this writing there is substantial research documenting the safety of some oils, and scant research about other oils.

Some of what we know about herbals and essential oils has been passed down through history. Before modern medicine, plants were the medicine. Indian and Chinese medicine have a tradition of using herbals that goes back hundreds of years. To a certain extent then, our knowledge of the uses and safety issues of essential oils comes to us from history and tradition. Some of the uses of essential oils have been extrapolated from the uses of their herbal counterpart in traditional medicine (e.g. if chamomile tea is relaxing then chamomile oil must also be relaxing). Fortunately, ongoing studies are being conducted in the modern era and are helping to either confirm or debunk what we know from traditional herbal medicine. We must bear in mind though that research and science are constantly evolving. What we once thought was fact has later been disproven (remember when margarine was better for us than butter?). Therefore I urge you to treat essential oils with the utmost respect because we may discover new information in the future that proves an oil unsafe. My recommendation is that just as you must follow dosage guidelines for medications such as acetaminophen or ibuprofen, you should use oils in moderation to prevent potential adverse effects. Remember that essential oils are much more concentrated than their herbal counterparts. The following rules should be observed:

1. **Never ingest essential oils.** Almost all of the documented serious events related to essential oils are due to ingestion. Some oils, such as eucalyptus, can be fatally toxic after ingesting just a milliliter or two. You will find sources that claim that if your oils are pure it is okay. Don't take any chances. The word "pure" on packaging labels is virtually meaningless. The exception to this rule is if a properly trained aromatherapist prescribes you an oil for ingestion. Even then, there are different schools of thought within the aromatherapy community regarding ingestion of essential oils and not all aromatherapists support ingestion.

I would like to propose that ingestion is the least effective way to benefit from essential oils. We have learned that topical application of oils to our skin results in them being absorbed into the skin, where they then enter the bloodstream. Inhalation of essential oils brings the molecules into our lungs where it is transferred from the alveoli into our bloodstream. When we ingest something it travels through our digestive system, where it is subject to digestive enzymes and the acidic environment of the stomach. Only once it has passed this gauntlet of gastric juices, which I might add are designed to break things down, does it reach the small intestine—the place where nutrients finally pass over into the bloodstream. Any substances that do not pass through into the blood are excreted as waste. I wonder whether essential oils make it as far as the small intestine without some change in their chemical makeup due to digestion? A scientist once told me that when we change a molecule's makeup, we change its properties. Regardless, because ingested oils need to make it to the small intestine before they can be absorbed, this will be the slowest method for getting essential oils into the bloodstream. Some food for thought, no pun intended.

2.   **Use caution with essential oils when you are pregnant.** There are only a handful of essential oils that are considered safe to use during pregnancy. Treat essential oils as if they were a drug (they are nature's medicine after all) and ask your doctor before using any essential oils. Remember that everything that enters your body finds its way into your baby's body, except he or she has a really tiny body so what may be a small dose for you is a large dose for your baby. Also remember that concrete safety data for essential oils used with pregnant mothers or children will be difficult to find. No one is going to be allowed to run a clinical trial to test for safety where a fetus or child is the test subject for fear of harming the child.

3.   **Avoid or exercise caution when using essential oils around small children and pets.** This is a rule that is oft-repeated but never very clearly defined. What is considered a small child? Most experts suggest that babies (over 6 months) and toddlers should not be exposed to any essential oils other than Lavender and Chamomile. While it is often suggested that children receive half of an adult dose, I think we can extrapolate some clearer guidance from conventional medicine. In medicine, a typical adult dose is usually based on a 150 lb adult so use this as a guideline when scaling dosages down for children. For example, a 75 lb child may receive a half dose, while a 50 lb child would receive one-third of a dose. When applying essential oils topically, this means adjusting the dilution rates. A 2% dilution for an adult would become a

1% dilution for a child. A 2% dilution would be 12 drops of essential oils into one ounce of base. The 75 lb child would therefore have 6 drops of essential oils per one ounce of base. The 50 lb child would have 4 drops per ounce of base. While weight is generally a more accurate way to adjust dosages for children, do factor in your child's age. There are fifty pound 3 year olds, and fifty pound 8 year olds. The three year old's organ maturity and ability to process and excrete the essential oil is not going to be the same as the eight year old. This is very important to remember as we cannot just treat children as mini-adults. (Think of all of the medications that we as adults take for granted that children shouldn't have until they are older).

We have looked at how to adjust dosages for topical administration, but that is not the focus of this book. How do we adjust dosages for children when we are diffusing essential oils? If you are using a diffuser where you mix essential oils with water you can adjust the concentration of oils that you add to the water. Just put a few less drops in the reservoir. The biggest concern will be the nebulizing diffuser, which propels a mist of pure undiluted essential oils into the environment (see Chapter 6 for an explanation of the different types of diffusers). I would suggest altering dosage with nebulizers by adjusting the time and frequency of diffusion.

Time—adjust the length of time that you run the diffuser. Instead of 10 minutes, run it for 5 minutes at a time. Also think about time of day. I run my nebulizing diffuser when my kids are in school or after they have gone to bed (in another part of the house). The molecules remain in the air for a few hours after the diffuser has been run so they still get the benefit without inhaling too much.

Frequency—the other variable you can alter is how often you run the diffuser. Instead of the usual two to three times a day for 10 minutes, you could run it 10 minutes once or twice a day.

Finally, only certain essential oils are considered safe for children. The Learning EO's website[5] has a nice chart of essential oils that can be used with children. The chart is based on the work of Robert Tisserand, who wrote the book (literally) on essential oil safety.

Certain pets, for example cats, are incapable of processing essential oils. If you have a pet and use a diffuser, make sure your pet is able to leave the room. Ask your vet or research which oils are safe for your pets.

4.   **Know your oils**. Research any oil that you plan to use paying particular attention to safety recommendations. Make sure your source is current. Books on aromatherapy that were published 20 years ago may contain different safety information than books that were published in recent years.   If using a web source, make sure it is up to date and unbiased. There are a lot of web sites that people have started with the best intentions but neglect to keep current.   There are also a lot of websites and personal blogs trying to sell you essential oils. Some contain misinformation so be wary.

There are some oils that should not be used yet are commercially available. A few examples include cinnamon bark, wintergreen and clove leaf. Several oils should be used with caution, for example cinnamon leaf and clove bud. If you have a medical condition pay particular attention to any oils with cautions for your condition.   Some oils that are high in phenols such as cinnamon or clove oil should not be used for more than 2 weeks at a time to avoid potential toxicity and overtaxing the liver. I list safety precautions for some of the most popular oils in Chapter 4.

5.   **Do not overuse essential oils**.   There are two common mentalities that I would like to address here:

"If a little is good, more is better" Not true with aromatherapy (and lots of other things!). Less is more when it comes to essential oils. Avoid the

temptation to put essential oils into your face cream, your lip balm, your body lotion, your soap, your diffuser, etc. It all adds up inside your body. If you do add essential oils to multiple products, take a minute to plan and add different oils to different products so you don't double and triple up the dosages of essential oils inadvertently. Studies have shown that essential oils have better effectiveness in small doses than larger ones.

"If it is natural, it is safe" Again, not true. Many natural products are not regulated by the FDA. These products *do not need to prove their safety or efficacy to be on the market.* Many plants in nature are poisonous or toxic. Others may provoke adverse or allergic reactions. Some cause sensitization reactions. Do not take for granted that a natural product is safe to use. Investigate the ingredients yourself or consult a qualified practitioner. Do a patch test to check for sensitivity.

6.   **Some essential oils are not compatible with some homeopathic treatments**.   If you use homeopathic treatments, consult your practitioner or check the oils you plan to use for contraindications.

7.   **Alternate essential oils**. Some oils should only be used for short periods of time. Alternate oils so you give your body a rest from the more potent oils. While microbes do not appear to grow resistant to essential oils, some aromatherapists feel it may not be a bad idea to give your body a break from a given oil so it does not grow accustomed to it thereby reducing effectiveness (Jones, 2014)[6].

8.   **Never allow undiluted essential oils to contact your skin or mucus membrane**s (examples of mucus membranes include the inside of your lips and mouth, eyes, and genital areas). Mucus membranes absorb substances much more rapidly than skin, which is thicker. Undiluted oils can cause sensitivity reactions, chemical burns, and allergic reactions. Never put essential oils on or near your eyes. If undiluted oils do contact your skin, you should apply a vegetable oil to the area and wipe it off with a tissue or towel. Repeat with more vegetable oil and then wash the area

with soap. If you are mixing your own blends, consider wearing gloves and protective eyewear. Re-cap essential oil bottles immediately to avoid accidental spills. Store essential oils out of the reach of children.

9.   **Do not substitute aromatherapy for seeking qualified medical advice**. It can be tempting to self-treat with essential oils however aromatherapy is considered a complementary therapy and you should treat it as such. If your condition requires the advice of a doctor or other qualified health practitioner, seek it. Use aromatherapy to supplement your health. As Marcel Lavabre put it, aromatherapy doesn't do your body's job, it helps your body do its job better.

If your medical condition is complex, again, get professional advice. When choosing an aromatherapist ask about their training and experience. There are many aromatherapy courses out there ranging from short self-study courses to one or two year programs in natural healing. Find an aromatherapist that has completed a program from a reputable provider whose coursework has sufficient breadth and depth. They should have studied the human body in health and disease as well as essential oils. Please note that in the United States, aromatherapists are not certified by any state or federal agency, so the term "certified aromatherapist" only means that they have completed some sort of program that issued a certificate of completion.

Chapter 4: Ten essential oils to get you started

When first purchasing essential oil there are two traps that are easy to fall into:

°Becoming so overwhelmed by choices that you don't know which oils to start with

°Or getting so excited that you end up with more bottles of essential oils than you know what to do with

Most essential oils have a shelf life of about one year so it is prudent to only buy what you need for up to a year at a time. In this section I share my top ten picks for getting started with diffusing essential oils. I chose many of these oils because they are so versatile in addressing a variety of complaints. Most of them have good safety profiles but a few of them are very potent and should be used only occasionally and with caution. I have included safety notes with each oil.

Sometimes people are disappointed with the lack of scent their diffuser produces. This can be the result of two different factors--the type of diffuser and the essential oil used. Some essential oils such as cinnamon have powerful aromas while others like lemon have mild aromas. For each of my top 10 oils I include the results of my own aroma testing. For each oil, I diffused it in a nebulizing diffuser--which provides the strongest scent, and a passive diffuser—which provides the weakest scent (see Chapter 6 for more about the types of diffusers). The results will give you an idea of how strong the aroma from each oil will be using each method. For all other diffuser types, you can expect the results to be somewhere in between as roughly indicated by this chart:

Strength of Aroma by Diffuser Type:

PASSIVE→PASSIVE/FAN→PASSIVE/HEAT→ULTRASONIC→NEBULIZER

Note: *Many of these oils have benefits beyond what I describe here.* Because this book is about diffusion, I have chosen to focus my discussion of each oil on the properties and benefits related to inhalation.

Lavender (Lavandula angustifolia, Lavandula officinalis)

Sources: France, Bulgaria, Hungary, Tasmania, Yugoslavia; the best quality lavender is considered to come from sources above 3000 feet

Extraction method: Steam distilled

Odor: Floral, herbaceous, and clean

Note: Top

Properties: Antiseptic, antidepressant, calming, harmonizing, immunostimulant, emmenagogue, decongestant

Uses: Anxiety, colds, coughs, depression, fatigue, flu, headaches, insect repellant, insomnia, nervousness, regulate menstrual flow, sinusitis, stress

Aroma Testing:

Oil Used: Lavandula officinalis (Hungary)

Passive (terracotta disc): Scent is barely discernible in a small room. May be suitable for a car diffuser or with aromatherapy jewelry.

Nebulizer: 10 minutes in a large room (open, high ceilings). After 10 minutes, there is a mild to moderate scent within 8 feet of the nebulizer. The scent is barely perceptible in the rest of the room. 10 minutes after turning it off the scent is barely perceptible.

Lavender has a history of use dating back to the Greeks. The Romans used it in their baths. During the 16th century it was used to fumigate sick rooms. Lavender has such a long list of beneficial properties that it is quite possibly the most versatile essential oil you can have in your collection. Lavender is known to be excellent for healing wounds such as burns and is suitable for a variety of skin complaints. In your diffuser, it is most useful for sedation, insomnia, nausea, headaches, depression, anxiety, antisepsis, and as an immune system stimulant.

Insomnia: Lavender is renowned for its relaxing effects so it is no surprise that it can help to promote restful sleep. According to Web M.D[7]. some studies have shown that vaporizing lavender overnight, or even just placing some on a gauze pad at bedside, may help people with mild insomnia. One very small study[8] at the University of Southampton in England found that 20% of subjects felt that they slept better in a lavender infused room versus a placebo. A slightly larger Korean study[9] of college women found that 60% felt an improvement in their sleep including such variables as length of time taken to fall asleep, severity of insomnia, and self-satisfaction with sleep. While these studies are small, they do suggest that lavender may be helpful in cases of mild insomnia.

Calming: One reason that lavender may work in promoting sleep is its sedative qualities. Lavender's sedative effects were demonstrated in a study[10] in which mice were injected with caffeine to induce hyperactivity and then exposed to lavender, which returned their activity levels to normal. Lavender can also be used to treat mild anxiety. A 2012 study[11] measured the response of participants to inhaled lavender oil versus a placebo base oil. Those that inhaled the lavender experienced reduced blood pressure, reduced heart rate and reduced skin temperature. This indicates a decrease in the arousal of the autonomic nervous system. The autonomic nervous system is connected to anxiety in that it is responsible for the fight or flight response. Usually a stressor will trigger the flight or fight response causing adrenalin to be released. After a period of time your body metabolizes adrenalin and returns to a normal state. In persons with anxiety, this normalization does not function properly. By decreasing arousal of the autonomic nervous system lavender may lessen the responses that lead to anxiety.

Immune stimulant: A healthy immune system is dependent on several factors including proper diet, regular exercise, and reduction of stress. We have already discussed Lavender's role in stress reduction. Robert Tisserand, in "Aromatherapy to Tend and Heal," states that lavender also stimulates both the production and activity of some types of white blood cells. White blood cells are an important part of the immune system, helping to attack foreign invaders such as viruses and bacteria. Lavender would therefore be excellent in a blend to promote everyday health as well as disease prevention.

Headaches and migraines: Lavender is promoted by most aromatherapists as useful for headaches. Indeed, many commercial essential oil blends for headaches contain lavender.   Despite this, scientific studies to back up this claim are scarce. One Iranian study[12] from 2012 did find promising results with migraine sufferers. Of 129 migraine sufferers who inhaled lavender oil, 71% reported partial or complete improvement of symptoms.   By contrast, 47% reported partial or complete improvement from inhaling a placebo.   These results are encouraging however given the high number who responded to placebos, similar studies should be conducted in order to confirm the findings.

There are many types of headaches (e.g. cluster, tension, migraine, etc.) and not all may respond equally well to lavender. I find that when you factor in lavender's ability to calm, reduce blood pressure, and its mild analgesic properties it definitely has a place in a headache blend. I recommend that you do your own experimentation though because for some, lavender *causes* a headache.

Insect repellant: Lavender is also noted as an insect repellant by many. Tisserand suggests that rather than being a repellant, it is most useful in the topical treatment of insect bites. I guess this means if the lavender doesn't keep the bugs away, you will at least have a way to neutralize the bites!

Lavender blends well with: Bergamot, Clary Sage, Geranium, Rosemary, Tea Tree, and any citrus oil

Safety: Lavender is generally considered to be a safe oil. Some people may have allergies or sensitivities to lavender and there are reports of nausea, vomiting and headache from inhalation or topical use of lavender. Topical use may also cause skin irritation in some. Because of its sedative effects, it may interact with other sedative medications such as CNS depressants (e.g. Ambien, Lorazepam), barbiturates (e.g. Amytal, Nembutal) and chloral hydrate (used for short term insomnia). If you are having surgery, you should ask your doctor if you should discontinue lavender use in the weeks leading up to surgery (Web MD)[7]. Some reports suggest that lavender may stimulate breast growth in young boys.

Lemon (Citrus Limon)

Sources: USA, Italy, South America

Extraction method: Cold pressed

Odor: Lemon

Note: Top

Properties: Antiseptic, disinfectant, immunostimulant, sedative, antidepressant, stimulant, antibacterial, antiviral, uplifting, decongestant, calming

Uses: Room disinfectant, immune stimulant, infectious diseases, depression, anxiety, fatigue, colds, flu, insomnia, mental concentration, clear the mind

Aroma Testing:

Oil Used: Citrus Limon-Organic (Italy)

Passive (terracotta disc): Minimal aroma detected

Nebulizer: After 10 minutes in a large room (open, high ceilings) a mild aroma is detected that fades quickly

----

Diffusing Lemon essential oil in your home will give it a mild, fresh, clean scent. It is also one of the best essential oils for air purification. As a bonus, you can also use it to create natural homemade cleaning products. Lemon is best known as being uplifting, an immune stimulant, and for its antiseptic properties.

Immune Stimulant: Like lavender, lemon oil is thought to stimulate white blood cells. This enhances the immune system. Some feel the immune stimulating properties of lemon oil are due to its high vitamin C content. It is true, lemon oil is expressed from lemon peel. Lemon peel provides 13% of your RDA for Vitamin C in 1 tablespoon (Self)[13] and it takes roughly 30 pounds of citrus to make 1 ounce of essential oil so you can imagine the concentration of Vitamin C. Because lemon oil is expressed from the peel where most pesticides accumulate, it is recommended that you buy organic lemon oil.

Aerial disinfection: Lemon oil is often added to cleaning products. It is easy to see why--it is a good disinfectant and it smells great. Pioneering aromatherapy researcher Dr. Jean Valnet reported that lemon vapors can kill Meningococcal bacteria in 15 minutes, Pneumococcal bacteria in less than 3 hours, and Staphylococcus aureus in 2 hours. Lemon essential oil can also kill typhus and diphtheria (from The Practice of Aromatherapy).

Mood Enhancing: Lemon oil smells refreshing so it is no surprise that it can positively affect mood. In 2008, a study[14] reported that inhaled lemon oil positively improved the mood of participants better than lavender or water. It also raised norepinephrine levels. Norepinephrine controls cognitive and emotional functions and is also involved in the fight or flight response. Too little norepinephrine can lead to depression, too much leads to anxiety, but normal levels can create a sense of well-being and euphoria (E-how)[15].

Lemon blends well with: Chamomile, Eucalyptus, Lavender, Geranium, Benzoin, Juniper, Sandalwood, and Fennel

Safety: Lemon oil may cause skin irritation if applied topically. Avoid sun or UV light when using lemon oil as it is phototoxic (increases your skin's susceptibility to damage from light).

Geranium (Pelargonium graveolens)

Sources: Europe, Egypt, China

Extraction method: Steam distilled

Odor: Floral, sweet

Note: Middle

Properties: Anti-depressant, sedative, antiseptic, uplifting, balancing, relaxing, anti-infectious

Uses: Insect repellant, PMS, depression, nervousness, menopause, fatigue, anxiety, depression, congestion, sore throat, stress

Aroma Testing:

Oil Used: Pelargonium Graveolens (Egypt)

Passive (terracotta disc): Moderate, lingering aroma. In a car, scent was detectable for 2 days.

Nebulizer: After 10 minutes in a large room (open, high ceilings) there is moderate aroma.

Geranium essential oil is a wonderful oil to have in your collection because not only does it provide emotional benefits when inhaled, but it can also be incorporated into skin care to promote cell regeneration and fade scars. In a diffuser, besides emotional benefits, it can be used as an antimicrobial.

Aerial Disinfection: In 2009, a study[2] found that a blend of Geranium and Lemongrass diffused in an office at 100% for 15 hours resulted in an 89% reduction in airborne bacteria. That is impressive! Now, the caveat is that most of us are not going to diffuse a blend for quite that long, but it does give some insight into the powerful antimicrobial effects of geranium as well as essential oils in general. Geranium has also been shown to inhibit MRSA (a form of staphylococcus aureus that is resistant to many antibiotics)[16]. Geranium blends well with other antimicrobial oils in this chapter such as clove, lemon, and rosemary.

Mood enhancing: Geranium is useful for nervousness and anxiety. It is considered to have a balancing effect on the emotions and tames tension. It may also lift the spirits in times of sadness.

Premenstrual Syndrome: Geranium is thought to balance hormones. It not only helps during PMS, but also other times of hormonal upheaval such as puberty and menopause. It can assist with some of the symptoms of PMS such as water retention and breast tenderness. Geranium's balancing properties can be useful in calming mood swings associated with PMS.

Geranium blends well with: Bergamot, Clary Sage, Lemon, Lavender, Rosemary, Clove, Chamomile, Grapefruit, Lime, and Peppermint

Safety: Geranium should not be used if you are pregnant. Geranium can cause skin irritation in some when applied topically.

Peppermint (Mentha piperita)

Sources: US, Europe

Extraction method: Steam distilled

Odor: Minty, fresh

Note: Top

Properties: Antiseptic, expectorant, uplifting, clearing, stimulant, expectorant, analgesic, decongestant, antibacterial

Uses: Headaches, mental clarity, fatigue, sinusitis, migraine, regulate menstrual flow, bronchitis, depression, nausea, motion sickness, insect repellant

Aroma Testing:

Oil Used: Peppermint Natural (Yakima) Mentha piperita

Passive (terracotta disc): In a small space, mild to moderate aroma

Nebulizer: After 10 minutes in a large room (open, high ceilings), there is a moderate fresh aroma that lingers for over an hour

---

Peppermint oil has been used for centuries. It is often recommended for digestive upsets as well as headaches. Peppermint is stimulating and can be used to improve mental focus and concentration. Peppermint has also been reported to be useful in repelling insects and mice.

Nausea and Motion Sickness: Peppermint oil is well known for aiding with nausea. Some clinical studies have found an improvement in post-operative nausea and vomiting (Tate, 1997)[17]. Another study (Jung & Lee, 2004)[18] found significantly lower nausea and vomiting with chemotherapy patients who inhaled peppermint oil. Peppermint may work by reducing "spasms in the digestive tract" (WebMD)[19]. In contrast, others have found that inhaling a placebo was equally effective in reducing nausea, suggesting it may be the focused breathing that brings relief (in order to gag you need to stop breathing momentarily). Peppermint may also help with motion sickness making it a useful oil to use in a car diffuser if you suffer from motion sickness.

Respiratory: Peppermint can be useful for treating respiratory conditions such as colds and flus. To treat a cough or nasal congestion, peppermint is often combined with eucalyptus oil. Warm steam can be helpful so diffusing oils in a bowl of steaming water can be therapeutic. An ultrasonic diffuser will provide cold humidity if you prefer. To take your therapy with you, a personal inhaler can be purchased or make one yourself by placing a few drops of your blend in a blank nasal inhaler (available online).

Headaches: Many people report relief from headaches after topical application of peppermint essential oil (properly diluted of course) to the temples. Peppermint may help to relieve headaches due to its analgesic

28

(pain relieving) effects or due to its vasodilating properties (opening the blood vessels, which increases blood flow).

Mental Focus: Inhalation of peppermint aroma has been found in multiple studies to improve memory and concentration. A 2006 study[20] of 144 participants found that peppermint aroma enhanced both memory and alertness when compared to the essential oil ylang-ylang and no aroma. Another study at the University of Cincinnati found that inhaling peppermint oil increased the accuracy of students taking a test by 28% (Dember, 1996). Other studies report increased memory by eating peppermint candies, however inhalation has fewer calories!

Peppermint blends well with: Rosemary, Eucalyptus, Lavender, Benzoin, Marjoram, Lemon, and Tea Tree

Safety: Despite its usefulness for treating headaches, inhaling peppermint too closely may cause headaches. Peppermint should not be used with children under 10 or during pregnancy. It can be a skin irritant so use caution if applying topically. This essential oil is not compatible with homeopathic therapy. Finally, due to its stimulating nature, it should not be used near bedtime.

Eucalyptus (Eucalyptus globulus)

Sources: Australia, Spain

Extraction: Steam distilled

Odor: Camphor, fresh, woody

Note: Top

Properties: Antiseptic, antiviral, decongestant, expectorant, disinfectant, antibacterial, stimulant

Uses: Insect repellant, break up mucus, bronchitis, flu, colds, sinusitis, headaches, mental fatigue, coughs, migraine, asthma, infectious diseases, improve concentration, mental clarity

Aroma Testing:

Oil Used: Eucalyptus globulus (Australia)

Passive (terracotta disc): Moderate aroma in a small room.

Nebulizer: 10 minutes in a large room (open, high ceilings). Mild to moderate aroma that fades within 30 minutes.

Eucalyptus oil comes from the leaves of the eucalyptus tree, a plant native to Australia. In aromatherapy, it has similar uses as peppermint oil in that is used for headaches, respiratory issues, repelling insects and improving mental concentration. Derivatives of eucalyptus oil are used in vapor rub cold formulas. There are several varieties of eucalyptus oil available and most aromatherapy books refer to Eucalyptus globulus unless otherwise specified. Other varieties include:

Eucalyptus radiata has similar properties to Eucalyptus globulus but is considered to be a safer oil. Marge Clark states
Eucalyptus radiata is less likely to trigger a cough reflex when inhaled. Kurt Schnaubelt considers it to be the best all-purpose eucalyptus oil.

Eucalyptus smithii is the mildest of the eucalyptus oils and the safest choice around children and the elderly (although avoid all eucalyptus around children under 10).

Eucalyptus citriodora has a lemony scent and can be used for respiratory conditions, air purification and as an insect repellant. While any eucalyptus can be used as an insect repellant, Eucalyptus citriodora (lemon eucalyptus) is the most frequently cited. It is part of a popular natural insect repellant sold by a major outdoor chain. There is some evidence that lemon eucalyptus may be more effective than the chemical insect repellant DEET.

Respiratory: One European study[21] suggested that eucalyptus' immune stimulating properties along with its antibacterial and antiviral activity make it effective in caring for respiratory infections. Indeed, many of the uses for eucalyptus relate to conditions such as bronchitis, asthma, colds, coughs, and sinus troubles. It can be used in a vaporizer as an expectorant for coughs. Its effectiveness is thought to result from its high eucalyptol content—averaging 70%. It breaks up mucus and so may be helpful for congestion. One effective way to use eucalyptus to relieve congestion is to place a few drops of the oil in a bowl of hot water and inhale the steam.

Headaches: Eucalyptus may help to relieve headaches and can be particularly helpful with sinus headaches. Be careful though, as too much eucalyptus may cause a headache. Eucalyptus is usually combined with other oils such as peppermint for treatment of headaches. One study[22] found that a blend of peppermint and eucalyptus had a muscle relaxant effect on headache sufferers, however peppermint alone provided the analgesic effect.

Eucalyptus blends well with: Benzoin, Lavender, Thyme, Lemon, Pine, Geranium, Peppermint, Rosemary

Safety: Avoid while pregnant and do not use with babies and young children (under 10). Small quantities can be fatal if ingested. Eucalyptus may not be compatible with homeopathic treatment.

Rosemary (Rosmarinus officinalis)

Sources: Mediterranean countries (Europe, Tunisia)

Extraction: Steam distilled

Odor: Strong, woody, camphor

Note: Middle

Properties: Antiseptic, analgesic, stimulant, anti-depressant, decongestant, anti-spasmodic

Uses: Mental stimulant, headache, fatigue, improve memory, alertness, depression, colds, bronchitis, flu, asthma, sinusitis, clear the mind, regulate menstrual flow

Aroma Testing:

Oil Used: Rosmarinus Officinalis (Morocco)

Passive (terracotta disc): Moderate in a small enclosed space

Nebulizer: After 10 minutes in a large room (open, high ceilings), moderate scent level that can be detected several feet away (10-12 feet)

Most of us are familiar with rosemary as a culinary herb. The essential oil is distilled from the flowering tops of the rosemary plant. In diffusion, it can be helpful to promote mental clarity, reduce fatigue, ease congestion from colds and sinusitis, and relieve headaches. Rosemary is a stimulating oil, so it should not be used at night or it may interfere with sleep.

There are two main chemotypes (varieties) of Rosemary essential oil:

Rosemary CT 1,8 cineol: Good for diffuser blends. Use for congestion, fatigue, stimulant, mental clarity, etc.

Rosemary CT verbenone: More commonly used in skin and hair care. May be useful for sinusitis.

When purchasing Rosemary, you should confirm with your supplier which variety of rosemary they carry.

Antimicrobial activity: In history, Rosemary was used for fumigations against the plague. In modern times, one study[23] found that rosemary oil had significant antimicrobial and antifungal activity against three bacteria and two fungi tested, including E.coli and Candida albicans. When combined with clove oil, the synergistic blend of the two oils produced even greater effects than either oil alone. This finding has been confirmed by other studies that have demonstrated both antibacterial and antifungal activity of rosemary essential oil.

Mental clarity: In the early half of the 1600's, English herbalist Nicholas Culpeper said of rosemary "It helpeth a weak memory, and quickeneth the senses." Rosemary is a stimulant and thus can be helpful in combatting mental fatigue as well as improving mental performance. Researchers have found that the aroma of rosemary essential oil increased memory and alertness in a series of mental tasks when compared to participants who inhaled lavender or no oil[24]. Another study[25] found a decrease in test taking anxiety among nursing students who inhaled lavender and rosemary essential oils. If you have a task that requires mental alertness consider diffusing rosemary oil.

Headaches: Rosemary is often recommended for headaches, and there are anecdotal reports of its particular effectiveness with migraines. This may be due to its ability to stimulate circulation. Migraines begin with a constriction of blood vessels in the brain followed by dilation of the vessels elsewhere in the body. Rosemary is thought to be tonic to the blood vessels which may explain its usefulness in easing migraines.

Rosemary blends well with: Basil, Cedarwood, Frankincense, Lavender, Peppermint, Geranium, Cinnamon, Eucalyptus, Tea tree, Lemon, Pine, and Ravensara

Safety: Do not use if you have high blood pressure, epilepsy, or are pregnant. Do not use with young children. Avoid using before bedtime or in large doses due to its stimulating effects. Topical use may irritate skin.

Tea Tree (Melaleuca alternifolia)

Sources: Australia

Extraction: Steam distilled

Odor: Sharp, fresh, woody, camphorous

Note: Middle

Properties: Antiseptic, expectorant, analgesic, antiviral, immunostimulant, decongestant, broad spectrum antimicrobial

Uses: Colds, bronchitis, immune stimulant, infectious diseases, flu, bronchitis, sinusitis **Aroma Testing**:

Oil Used: Melaleuca alternifolia (Australia) Organic

Passive (terracotta disc): Mild to moderate in a small enclosed space

Nebulizer: After 10 minutes in a large room (open, high ceilings), there is a moderately strong scent that lingers several minutes after turning it off. Scent can be detected several feet away.

My first introduction to tea tree oil was when the Body Shop® released an acne care line based on tea tree. I had no idea back in the 90's how many other powerful properties this oil had. Tea tree is native to Australia where it has been used by aboriginal people for years. It is known as an anti-infective and immune stimulant. In a diffuser it is also recommended for respiratory conditions.

Immune stimulant: Tea tree is one of the more powerful oils with immune stimulating properties. Julia Lawless states that tea tree increases the body's ability to respond to pathogens. In one study[26], mice inhaling tea tree oil experienced an increase in circulating immunoglobulins, as well as other immune system cells. In aromatherapy references, tea tree is one of the most cited oils for increasing immune system activity.

Antimicrobial: There is some debate among the scientific community as to whether tea tree is the superstar antimicrobial that the herbal community claims it to be. This is due in part to a lack of studies proving its effectiveness. Most research about tea tree focuses on topical use of tea tree for skin infections. Despite this, two studies[27] of vaporized tea tree oil showed it to have some effect against bacteria. The first study found that organisms such as E. coli, H. influenzae, S. pyogenes (strep throat) and S. pneumonia were inhibited by vaporized tea tree oil. A second study described reports of a reduction in hospital acquired infections due to vaporized tea tree oil. Tea tree is one essential oil thought to be effective against viruses, bacteria, and fungi.

Respiratory diseases: Breathing in the vapors of tea tree can be useful for loosening phlegm when you have sinus congestion or a cold. Because it is a decongestant and expectorant, it will also aid in other respiratory conditions such as bronchitis and coughs. Besides loosening mucus, the antiviral effects may help to fight the cold virus itself. To use for respiratory conditions, you may wish to blend it with other useful respiratory oils such as eucalyptus or peppermint.

Tea tree blends well with: Eucalyptus, Lavender, Juniper, Lemon, Rosemary, Thyme, German Chamomile, Clary sage, Clove, Geranium

Safety: May be a skin irritant and/or a skin sensitizer. Never take internally as it can be toxic.

Chamomile (Anthemis nobilis; Matricaria chamomilla)

Roman Chamomile (Anthemis nobilis, Chamaemelum nobile)

German Chamomile (Matricaria chamomilla, Chamomilla recutita)

Sources: Europe, USA

Extraction: Steam distilled

Odor: Herbal, strong, sweet

Note: Middle

Properties: Immunostimulant, antidepressant, sedative, emmenagogue, antiseptic, analgesic, anti-inflammatory

Uses: Nervousness, headaches, immune stimulant, insomnia, migraines, irritability, tantrums, stress, anxiety, anger, menstrual regulation

Aroma Testing:

Oil Used: Matricaria Chamomilla (Egypt)

Passive (terracotta disc): In a small enclosed space, there is a strong scent that lingers

Ultrasonic: Due to the high cost of Chamomile, I tested this one in an ultrasonic diffuser under the same conditions—large, open room with high ceilings. Within minutes there was moderately strong aroma within a few feet of the machine and a mild aroma several feet away.

Chamomile is the queen of calm. It has been used in Europe for centuries for medicinal purposes. Think of the relaxation a cup of chamomile tea provides and you will know why it is a popular essential oil for treating nervousness, insomnia, and stress. Chamomile has a strong smell that reminds me of hay. Use chamomile sparingly as in addition to being costly, you can easily overpower a blend with it.

There are two varieties of chamomile, Roman and German. German chamomile essential oil has a deeper blue color due the presence of the anti-inflammatory component azulene. The blue color will fade over time to yellow. Roman chamomile essential oil has a pale blue color. *When it comes to aromatherapy, both have similar effects.* The main difference is the two oils come from different species of plant.

Calming: Chamomile is a powerful sedative and can help to reduce nervous tension and calm anger. Chamomile can be used around toddlers so it may help to "diffuse" temper tantrums, or make children sleepy. Remember to always reduce dosages around children. Use it in the evening to unwind from a stressful day and prepare yourself for sleep. Not only is it calming to the mind, but if you make your own skin care products the anti-inflammatory compounds in this oil can help to calm your skin as well.

Headaches and migraines: Chamomile's sedative and antiinflammatory properties make it another oil that may help in a headache blend. It is not one of the most common headache oils, but rather, add it to a blend of oils such as peppermint, rosemary or lavender. Peppermint and rosemary can be very stimulating oils but some headaches are stress and tension related. Adding a drop or two of chamomile to your headache blend can ease the tension behind the headache.

Premenstrual syndrome: Chamomile is thought to be balancing to the female reproductive system. It may stimulate menstrual flow and help to ease cramps. Blend it with lavender, geranium or clary sage to create your own PMS solution.

Chamomile blends well with: Lavender, Bergamot, Geranium, Lemon, Orange, Ylang Ylang, Clary Sage, Patchouli, Tea tree, and Grapefruit

Safety: Avoid if pregnant. May cause skin irritation

Clove Bud (Eugenia caryophyllata)

Sources: Indonesia, Madagascar

Extraction: Steam distilled

Odor: Spicy, warm, cloves

Note: Middle

Properties: Analgesic, antiseptic, aphrodisiac, stimulant, broad spectrum antibacterial, antiviral

Uses: Sinusitis, improve memory, infectious diseases, bronchitis, fatigue

Aroma Testing:

Oil Used: Eugenia Caryophyllata (Indonesia)

Passive (terracotta disc): Mild aroma in a small enclosed space

Nebulizer: After 10 minutes in a large room (open, high ceilings), there is a mild aroma that lingers for up to 30 minutes.

_____

Clove bud essential oil is a powerful oil and must be used with caution. Be aware that there is also a Clove leaf oil which should never be used.

Clove oil is included in this list because of its inclusion in several antimicrobial blends, including the popular Thieves® oil. Clove oil has strong antioxidant properties and can also be used for respiratory diseases, as an insect repellant, and as an aphrodisiac.

Antibacterial/Room purification: Clove oil is a broad spectrum antibacterial and antiviral (Schnaubelt, Advanced Aromatherapy). In a diffuser, it can be useful to purify the air and room of bacteria and viruses. During the bubonic plague, it was one of the oils/herbs that grave robbers claimed kept them from getting sick while scavenging the graves of infected bodies. If you want to make your own version of Thieves® oil you will need a small bottle of this oil in your arsenal.

Mental Fatigue: Clove oil is a mentally stimulating oil and helps to counteract fatigue and lethargy. It is also thought to stimulate memory. In a diffuser it is pleasantly warming and blending it with cinnamon and orange is a popular combination for a feel good pick me up.

Clove Bud blends well with: Chamomile, Clary Sage, Geranium, Grapefruit, Lavender, Cinnamon, Rose, Rosemary, and Bergamot

Safety: Never use Clove leaf oil, only Clove bud oil. Clove bud oil contains eugenol, which is a phenol. Essential oils high in phenols should not be used in large doses or for extended periods of time as it could cause liver damage. Do not use Clove oil for more than two weeks at a time. Do not apply directly to skin or mucous membranes as it can be irritating. Do not use if you have liver or kidney disease. Do not use around young children or during pregnancy. Dr. Robert Tisserand also recommends not using clove oil if you suffer from alcoholism, hemophilia, prostrate cancer, and anticoagulant therapy. Can be sensitizing.

Cinnamon leaf (Cinnamomum zeylanicum)

Sources: Ceylon, India, China, Madagascar

Extraction: Steam distilled

Odor: Warm, spicy, cinnamon

Note: Middle

Properties: Antiseptic, stimulant, aphrodisiac

Uses: Colds, flu, infectious diseases, irregular menstruation, nervous exhaustion, stress

Aroma Testing:

Oil Used: Cinnamomum Zeylanicum (Sri Lanka)

Passive (terracotta disc): Moderate strength in a small enclosed space

Nebulizer: After 10 minutes in a large room (open, high ceilings) there is a moderate aroma throughout the room

---

Cinnamon is one of my favorite oils in a blend as it has a warm, spicy smell that blends wonderfully with orange oil. Due to its high phenol content it should be used in low concentrations and for no more than 2 weeks at a time, so alas I can't use it all the time! There are two varieties of Cinnamon oils available: Cinnamon Bark and Cinnamon Leaf. Each are extracted from a different part of the cinnamon plant as their names suggest. Cinnamon Bark oil should never be used. Cinnamon Leaf oil can be a skin sensitizer but is the safer of the two oils. Cinnamon is another of the ingredients in blends based on the thieves' legend.

Aerial disinfection: When blended with other oils such as clove, lemon, tea tree, rosemary or geranium, you can create a powerful aerial disinfectant. An article[28] published in the Journal of Complementary and Alternative Medicine found that even at low concentrations Cinnamon was a good inhibitor of bacteria. Other research supports this finding. Because of safety concerns in using oils high in phenols such as Cinnamon and Clove I reserve these oils for times when there is an active illness in the house or after a known exposure to an illness. Other antiseptic oils should be used for everyday disinfection and I recommend rotating through a few different oils such as Lemon, Tea tree, Rosemary, Geranium and Ravensara for aerial disinfection.

Colds & Flus: Cinnamon can be useful against colds and flus as well as other short term viruses. It has potent antiviral and antibacterial actions and is also helpful for symptoms such as coughs. In addition, I find it gives a pleasant, warming sensation which is comforting when you have a cold or chills.

Cinnamon Leaf blends well with: Benzoin, Clove, Frankincense, Ginger, Grapefruit, Peppermint, and Rosemary

Safety: Never use Cinnamon Bark oil. Use sparingly as it can be an irritant and sensitizer. Can cause skin irritation. Avoid if pregnant. Tisserand also recommends avoiding with certain cancers, kidney and liver disease, alcoholism, hemophilia, and anti-coagulant therapy. Lavabre cautions it may cause convulsions in high doses.

Eleven more oils that work well in a diffuser

Bergamot (Citrus bergamia): Bergamot is a top note with a floral, citrusy aroma. If you have ever had earl grey tea, you know the scent of bergamot. It is useful for stress, anxiety and tension—helping to balance and uplift. Its expectorant properties make it useful in blends for colds and its antiseptic properties may help to disinfect the air. Bergamot can also be sedative and therefore useful for insomnia.

Bergamot is a wonderful oil to have on hand in that it blends well with a variety of oils.

Safety: Can be phototoxic (make your skin more sensitive to light), you can avoid this by selecting FCF versions of bergamot.

Cedarwood (Cedrus atlantica): Cedarwood has a balsamic, woody scent. As a base note, it is useful as a fixative in blends, however is too thick for use in nebulizing diffusers. Marcel Lavabre suggests it can serve as a substitute for Sandalwood due to their similar emotional effects (Sandalwood is both expensive and endangered). It can be used in blends for air purification, coughs, stress, anxiety, and for repelling insects.

Safety: Do not use on children under 10. Avoid if pregnant. May cause skin irritation.

Citronella (Cymbopogon nardus): Citronella may be familiar to you from the citronella candles burned to repel insects. Indeed, one of the uses of the essential oil is as an insect repellant. It is a top note with a fresh, lemony scent. Citronella can be used for even smaller pests—it is useful in disinfecting a room from germs.

Safety: Avoid if pregnant. May cause skin irritation.

Clary Sage (Salvia sclarea): Clary sage is a middle note with a floral, musky scent. Among its many uses are relief from stress, anxiety and depression. It is also useful with PMS, menopause, and menstrual difficulties. It is considered an aphrodisiac and can cause euphoria.

Safety: Do not confuse clary sage with common sage, which is unsafe to use. Do not use while driving or consuming alcohol. Do not use if pregnant.

Frankincense (Boswellia carteri): Frankincense is a base note oil whose aroma can be described as balsamic, woody, camphorous and citrusy. Often used in religious ceremonies, it can be calming and grounding which also makes it good for meditation. It is a useful oil for respiratory conditions such as colds and bronchitis due to its expectorant qualities. The oil is too thick to use in a nebulizer.

Safety: No precautions reported.

Juniper (Juniperus communis): This middle note oil has a fruity, woody scent and can help to disinfect the air. It can be used for coughs, colds, and flu. Emotionally, it can ease stress and promote mental clarity.

Safety: Use sparingly. Do not use if you are pregnant, or have liver or kidney disease.

Myrrh (Commiphora myrrha): Myrhh is a base note oil with a warm, balsamic, musty scent. Like Frankincense, it is a thick oil that is not suitable for nebulizers. It promotes emotional well-being and is useful in spiritual practices. It is also antiviral and particularly useful for respiratory conditions such as coughs, colds, and bronchitis.

Safety: Do not use during pregnancy. Use in low concentrations due to possible toxicity. Never ingest myrrh due to its toxicity.

Petitgrain (Citrus aurantium): Petitgrain comes from the leaves and twigs of the same plant that Neroli and Orange oil come from. It has a woody, floral, citrus scent and is a top note. Petitgrain is wonderful for emotional conditions such as stress, mental fatigue, anxiety, and nervousness. It is also used for insomnia and to stimulate memory.

Safety: No precautions noted

Pine (Pinus sylvestris): Pine is a middle note with a fresh scent like a forest and makes a good natural air freshener. Pine can be used for respiratory conditions such as colds, sinusitis, coughs, and flu. It may also help with hangovers.

Safety: Possible skin irritant/sensitizer

Ravensara (Ravensara aromatic): Ravensara is a less well known oil that has good anti-viral properties. It is a top note with an herbal, camphorous scent. Use it to help with viral diseases such as flu and colds. It is also an immune system stimulant.

Safety: Do not use during pregnancy. Limited safety data available.

Ylang Ylang (Cananga odorata): Ylang ylang is a love it or hate it oil. It has a very sweet, floral scent and can be a middle or a base note. There are several varieties available and those labelled extra or complete are considered the best for aromatherapy. Ylang ylang is an aphrodisiac. It can also be used for a host of emotional issues such as depression, stress, and anxiety as well as balancing emotions in general.

Safety: Do not use during pregnancy. High doses may cause headaches, nausea or euphoria.

Chapter 5: Essential Oils Used in Healing

This chapter looks at several common ailments and pairs them with recommended oils. While every effort has been made to include our top 10 oils, at times a condition is better served by other oils. After all, there are over 300 essential oils. This section looks at the *best* oils for each condition. As choosing scents can be personal, I don't give too many recipes, but rather give you the tools to experiment with your own blending. To get you started, let's go over a few tips on blending.

Creating your own blends—"notes" on blending

Creating your own blend is part science, part art, and part personal preference.

The science of blending relates to choosing the appropriate oils for the intended effect. For example, if you are blending for a stress busting effect, you will need to choose oils that are known to alleviate stress. When blended, some oils work together to create a greater effect than the sum of their parts. 1+1=3. This is called synergy. Synergy is a bit magical in that it is difficult to predict. I liken it to music: there can be a whole host of mediocre bar bands but every once in a while the right combination of people making music is out of this world. There is no way to know what that right combination of musicians may be, you just need to keep trying until you get it right— and when its right you will know! That said, as beginning blenders a general rule of thumb is to limit your blends to 3 oils. Remember that less is more and you don't want to overcomplicate your blend.

The art of blending is much like the art of the perfumer. Choosing top, middle and base notes will help you to achieve balanced blends. Top notes hit your nose first, but dissipate quickly. Base notes are not immediately noticed, but provide a scent that will linger and can help to fix the lighter notes. The middle notes help to balance the two. Perfumers use notes when blending. While not imperative, using the notes to guide your blend can help you to achieve a harmonious blend more easily.

Your very first blends should start with three oils, preferably a base, middle, and top note. For a 10 drop blend, start with 2 drops of your base note oil. Then add 3-5 drops of your middle note oil, and finish it off with 3-5 drops of your top note oil. The next step is to let it sit for a day. This helps the fragrances to marry with each other. Apply a little to a cotton swab the next day and take a sniff. Adjust the proportions according to your tastes. Be sure to keep notes of what oils you used and how many drops of each. If you hit upon that perfect blend you want to be able to replicate it! Do note that not all blends in this book or elsewhere include a base note oil, but including one when possible will help your scent to linger longer.

The final aspect of blending is personal preference. Art and science mean nothing if it does not smell good to you. Your blend should be pleasing to you. Use the sniff test described above and keep experimenting!

Essential Oils for Health and Wellness:

Essential oils can be used for both physical and emotional wellness. This can be a wonderful boon to ease everyday illnesses and to help with life's ups and downs. It bears repeating that you should seek the advice of a qualified health professional for any physical, mental, or emotional ailment that requires treatment. The best use of aromatherapy is not to self-treat, but as complementary therapy. Complementary therapy, as defined by the National Center for Complementary and Alternative

Medicine, is the use of non-mainstream approaches alongside conventional medicine. The essential oils and blends discussed in this section will give you some ideas as to how aromatherapy can assist with common complaints. I have placed in bold type the oils that are part of your beginner's oil toolkit from Chapter 4.

Colds & Sinuses

Colds are no fun but we all seem to get one or two a year, especially if you have children in your life. Colds are caused by viruses and usually affect the upper respiratory tract. Common symptoms include coughing, sneezing, runny or stuffy nose, and sore throat. The good news is while conventional medicine can help you *feel* better, by easing the symptoms, essential oils may help you *heal* by attacking the virus—the root cause. This is a perfect example of conventional and alternative medicine working hand in hand. I can attest that since I began diffusing essential oils, my family has experienced fewer colds. When someone does get sick, it is usually quite mild and they recover quickly. Essential oils are not only anti-viral, but many are known for helping with specific cold symptoms such as coughing or congestion. The following oils can be helpful in preventing and treating a cold.

Strengthen the Immune System: **Lavender, Lemon, Tea Tree**, Pine, Ravensara, Eucalyptus, Bergamot, and Frankincense

Coughs: **Eucalyptus, Lavender, Rosemary, Tea Tree, Peppermint**, Cypress, and Frankincense

Runny Nose: **Eucalyptus, Lemon, Lavender, Peppermint**, Cypress

Sore Throat: **Lavender, Lemon, Eucalyptus, Peppermint**, Thyme, Cypress

Top recommended oils for a cold (general) by note:

Top: **Eucalyptus, Lavender, Peppermint, Lemon**, Ravensara, Basil

Middle: **Rosemary, Tea Tree**, Pine, Cypress, Marjoram, Black Pepper

Base: Benzoin, Frankincense

Sample Blends

Cold Blend #1: 6 drops Eucalyptus, 6 drops Lemon and 4 drops Tea Tree

Cold Blend #2: 3 drops Rosemary, 2 drops Peppermint, 3 drops Lavender

Cough Blend: 1 drop Frankincense, 2 drops Lavender, 2 drops Eucalyptus

Flus & Viruses

Another common viral infection is the flu. Flu symptoms can be similar to cold symptoms but also cause body aches, fever, chills, headache, and sometimes nausea, vomiting and diarrhea. Each year, vaccinations are available for the strains that experts predict will be the worst for that year, but it is not protection from all flus. There are many strains and viruses mutate often. Many of the same oils that combat cold viruses will also help with flu viruses.

Strengthen the Immune System: **Lavender, Lemon, Tea Tree**, Pine, Ravensara, **Eucalyptus**, Bergamot, and Frankincense

Headaches: **Lavender, Peppermint, Chamomile, Rosemary, Marjoram**

Nausea: **Peppermint, Lavender**, Black Pepper, Ginger, Nutmeg, Patchouli

Top recommended oils for flu (general) by note:

Top: **Eucalyptus, Lavender, Peppermint, Lemon**, Ravensara

Middle: **Rosemary, Cinnamon, Tea Tree**, Black pepper, Cypress

Sample Blends

Anti-viral blend #1: 2 drops Tea Tree, 2 drops Ravensara, 2 drops Lemon, 1 drop Eucalyptus

Anti-viral blend #2 (based on thieves legend): 2 drops Rosemary, 2 drops Lemon, 1 drop Cinnamon Leaf, 1 drop Clove Bud, 2 drops Eucalyptus.

Everyday viral prevention: 3 drops Lavender, 2 drops Geranium

Immune Boosting: 4 drops Lemon, 3 drops Tea Tree, 2 drops Lavender

Headaches

Headaches can put a crimp in your day, while migraines can flatten you. For everyday headaches, essential oils can be an alternative to popping a pain pill. For migraine sufferers, it may be used as complementary therapy. Besides migraines, there are cluster headaches and tension headaches. Some headaches are secondary to another condition such as flu, sinus problems, dehydration and many other causes. If your headache is worse than usual or presents with unusual symptoms such as high fever, slurred speech, stiff neck, confusion, paralysis, etc., you should consult a doctor immediately. For common headaches, try these essential oils:

Migraines: **Peppermint, Rosemary, Lavender**, Basil, Marjoram

Sinus Headaches: **Eucalyptus, Peppermint**

Top recommended oils for headaches (general) by note:

Top: **Lavender, Peppermint, Lemon, Eucalyptus**, Basil

Middle: **Roman Chamomile, Rosemary**, Marjoram, Bay, Rosewood

Sample Blends

Headache Blend: 4 drops Peppermint, 2 drops Rosemary, 4 drops Lavender

Migraine Blend: 3 drops Marjoram, 2 drops Lavender, 1 drop Peppermint

Nausea and Motion Sickness

Nausea is usually a symptom of some underlying disease or condition. It can be caused by viruses, medications, or other diseases. Motion sickness is an inner ear disturbance caused by repeated motion such as riding in a boat, car, or airplane. Motion sickness can cause nausea that may lead to vomiting. Essential oils may help to treat or prevent nausea and motion sickness. If you are susceptible to motion sickness, you may try diffusing a blend from the oils below in a car diffuser. If you believe your nausea is viral, consider including immune stimulating and antiviral oils (see Flu above) such as Lavender, Tea Tree, Rosemary or Cinnamon.

Top recommended oils for nausea and motion sickness by note:

Top: **Peppermint, Lavender**, Basil

Middle: Black Pepper, Ginger (can also be a base note)

Base: Patchouli

Sample Blend

Nausea Blend: 2 drops Peppermint, 2 drops Lavender, 2 drops Ginger

Insomnia

One of the most popular oils for relaxation is Lavender, however there are other oils that can help you get a good night's sleep. Diffusing is a great way to use essential oils for insomnia as it is a hands free method of administration. You can place a few drops on a tissue or other passive diffuser at your bedside, or set a timer on your ultrasonic device to diffuse a gentle aroma into your bedroom intermittently throughout the night.

Top recommended oils for insomnia by note:

Top: **Lavender**, Bergamot,

Middle: **Roman Chamomile**, Clary Sage, Marjoram, Ylang ylang (can also be base)

Base: Sandalwood

Sample Blends

Insomnia blend #1: 6 drops Lavender, 6 drops Bergamot, 2 drops Roman Chamomile

Insomnia blend #2: 4 drops Lavender, 4 drops Clary Sage, 2 drops Roman Chamomile

Stress Relief and Relaxation

For all the tools and services we have in our modern world to make our lives easier, we seem to be more stressed and life is more hectic than ever. Relaxation is an important part of maintaining health and we should all take time daily to relax and decompress from the day. Stress can cause a multitude of symptoms including weight changes, sleep disturbances, heart palpitations, nausea and diarrhea to name just a few. Stress relief begins with identifying potential stressors in your life—major life changes, work, school, family issues, etc. and taking steps to avoid the stressor, or change your response to it. Engaging in exercise and relaxing activities like a hobby can help to let off some of the tension of stress. Practices such as yoga, meditation, or tai chi may also help take your mind away from stressors. Diffusing essential oils can help to set the atmosphere for taking a relaxing time out.

Top recommended oils for stress and relaxation by note:

Top: **Lavender**, Bergamot

Middle: **Chamomile, Geranium**, Ylang Ylang (can also be a base note), Clary Sage, Neroli, Palmarosa, and Rose

Base: Patchouli, Sandalwood

Sample Blends

Stress blend #1: 2 drops Lavender, 3 drops bergamot, 2 drops Clary Sage

Stress blend #2: 2 drops Chamomile, 2 drops Geranium, 1 drop Ylang Ylang, 3 drops Lavender

Uplifting and Stimulating Oils

Ever need a pick me up during the day that doesn't involve another cup of coffee? Essential oils may be the answer. The wonderful thing is that many of the citrus family oils are uplifting so diffusing them will make your home smell fresh and you'll feel great! Many citrus oils are top notes so they evaporate quickly, but adding a bit of Litsea cubeba (also known as May Chang) as a fixative can help to anchor your blend. Litsea cubeba has a citrusy aroma and is a balancing and uplifting oil in its own right.

Rosemary is another stimulating oil. In fact, it is so stimulating that you should not use this oil before bedtime. Rosemary has the added benefit of increasing mental clarity, making you feel both physically and mentally charged. Similarly, peppermint oil has the dual benefit of both mental and physical stimulation. A whiff of peppermint is refreshing and bracing. Clove oil is stimulating and energizing. It is a potent oil however, and should only be used for no more than two weeks at a time.

Top recommend oils to uplift and stimulate by note:

Top: **Lemon, Peppermint**, Grapefruit, Lime

Middle: **Clove, Rosemary**, Litsea Cubeba (May Chang)

Sample Blends

Uplifting Blend #1: 3 drops Grapefruit, 2 drops Lemon, 2 drops Litsea Cubeba

Uplifting Blend #2: 6 drops Grapefruit, 3 drops Clove Bud, 1 drop Peppermint

Anxiety

Anxiety is a real and debilitating condition. True anxiety goes beyond feeling a little nervous and the sufferer may have panic attacks, palpitations or other physical manifestations. Reassurance will not be enough to alleviate anxiety and sometimes a person is incapable of coping with life's stresses without medication. If your symptoms match this description, you should consult a health practitioner. Aromatherapy may bring relief to mild anxiety, or serve as a complementary therapy in more severe cases.

Top recommended oils for anxiety by note:

Top: **Lavender**, Bergamot, and Petitgrain

Middle: **Chamomile, Geranium**, Ylang ylang, Neroli, Jasmine, Rose, Marjoram

Base: Frankincense, Benzoin, Patchouli

Sample Blends

Anxiety Blend #1: 3 drops Lavender, 1 drop Chamomile, 2 drops Bergamot

Anxiety Blend #2: 1 drop Frankincense, 6 drops Lavender, 4 drops Geranium

Depression

Depression is likely to affect all of us at some point in our lives. For most of us it is short term, but in others it can become a chronic issue. It can have physical implications such as loss of appetite, mood swings, and anxiety. Depressed persons may shun social activities. (Recently, centenarians were interviewed, and one common factor of these long lived souls was their friendships and social ties). If you have chronic depression, are depressed for more than a few days, or entertain thoughts of harming yourself you should consult your health practitioner. The following essential oils can be an adjunct therapy for the chronically depressed, or short term therapy for the occasional down days.

Top recommended oils for depression by note:

Top: **Lavender, Lemon**, Bergamot,

Middle: **Geranium, Chamomile**, Jasmine, Rose, Ylang ylang, Clary Sage, Neroli,

Base: Frankincense, Patchouli

Sample Blends

Depression Blend #1: 2 drops Bergamot, 2 drops Lemon, 1 drop Clary Sage, 1 drop Frankincense

Depression Blend #2: 2 drops Lavender, 4 drops Geranium, 2 drops Lemon

Mental Alertness and Concentration

There are some days when you need to focus on a job or assignment and you just can't get your head in the game. Good sleep is essential to concentration and if sleep is an issue, consider using aromatherapy at night for insomnia (see Insomnia above). During the daytime, essential oils can improve memory, concentration and alertness. One study[29] published in 2013 found that test subjects that inhaled rosemary were able to remember 60-75% more of their assigned tasks than those in a control group (no scent).

Top recommended oils for mental alertness and concentration by note:

Top: **Peppermint, Lemon**, Basil, Bergamot

Middle: **Rosemary, Clove**, Black Pepper, Juniper

Sample Blends

Concentration Blend #1: 2 drops lemon, 2 drops rosemary

Concentration Blend #2: 3 drops rosemary, 2 drops peppermint, 1 drop Clove Bud

Essential oils for the car

There are a few diffusers on the market designed for use in your car. These can be used to freshen your car with natural scents but because some essential oils can be sedative, care must be taken to avoid oils that may make you drowsy or lose focus. Any of the oils used for mental alertness and concentration would be great for use in your car. If you are prone to road rage, you may want to add a drop or two of Lavender to a blend of more stimulating oils. Never use clary sage or marjoram when driving as they can be sedating.

Top recommended oils for driving by note:

Top: **Lemon, Lavender, Peppermint**

Middle: **Rosemary**

Sample Blend

Driving Blend: 3 drops Rosemary, 3 drops Lemon and 1 drop Lavender

Chapter 6: Choosing a diffuser

With aromatherapy enjoying a surge in popularity right now, the number of diffusers on the market has increased greatly in recent years. It can be confusing to decide which one is the right one for you. The right one, of course, will be different for everyone. Factors include:

°The size of the space it is being used for

°The purpose of diffusing essential oils (e.g. scent/mood, therapeutic benefits, or both)

°How much maintenance the diffuser requires

°Whether it will it be used around small children or pets

As we discuss the different types of diffusers we will be addressing these factors. Diffusers can be divided into two main categories: active and passive. Active diffusers use a pump or ultrasonic technology that helps to break up and propel the essential oil into the air. Active diffusers do not heat up the oils. Heat is a bad thing because it is thought to destroy or alter the therapeutic properties of essential oils. Passive diffusers work via simple evaporation. Some passive diffusers use a fan to promote evaporation and blow the aromatic molecules further into the room. Other passive devices use heat to speed evaporation of the oil. The biggest drawback to passive devices is that the chemical components making up the essential oil may evaporate at different rates, possibly changing the therapeutic benefits of the oil. Essential oils are made up of various molecules (e.g. thymol, eugenol, etc.). If one type of molecule evaporates faster than the others, the proportions change and we end up with an altered oil. To illustrate this, think of chocolate chip cookies—altering the amount of sugar or flour will make the cookie more chewy or crispy.

Types of Active Diffusers

Active diffusers are considered more therapeutic than passive diffusers and include models that are labeled or described as nebulizers and ultrasonic.

Nebulizers

Nebulizers take pure, undiluted essential oil and break it into a fine mist that is propelled into the air. They are usually powered by an aquarium pump or similar device which can cause a low hum during use. This is the biggest complaint people have about nebulizers aside from the cost, which is among the highest of all types of diffusers.

Advantages of Nebulizing Diffusers:

°No heat is used. Heat can alter the properties of essential oils by hastening the evaporation of some of the components

°The particles released into the air are fine enough to remain suspended in the air for a few hours after use

°Uses undiluted essential oil

°Can quickly fill a space with aroma, with some units capable of covering a large area

°Can "clean" the air of bacteria, viruses, and fungi as well as inhibit bacterial growth on surfaces in the room

°Highly fragrant due to the concentration of oil released

Disadvantages of Nebulizing Diffusers:

°Some units emit a low hum during use, noise is usually proportional to output level

°Devices cannot be used with thick essential oils such as Frankincense or Myrrh as they will clog the device

°Devices cannot be used with essential oils that have been mixed with carrier oils

°Oils left sitting in the unit for long periods may thicken (due to evaporation) and clog the device

°Requires periodic cleaning

°Cost is usually higher than other types of diffusers

Ultrasonic Diffusers

Ultrasonic diffusers also disperse fine particles of essential oil into the air. Because the essential oil is placed into a reservoir of water, the resultant mist is less concentrated than nebulizers. This can be a benefit if you do not want a strong concentration of oils.

Advantages of Ultrasonic Diffusers

°Less concentrated mist than a nebulizer (may be an advantage or a disadvantage depending on your requirements)

°No heat is used so properties of essential oils are not altered

°Quieter than a nebulizer

°Adds moisture to the air (humidifies) which may be an advantage or disadvantage depending on how dry or wet your climate is

°Some devices may tolerate thicker oils, check with the manufacturers recommendations

°Many have timers, intermittent cycles and/or automatic shutoff when the unit runs out of water

Disadvantages of Ultrasonic Diffusers

°Less concentrated oil is dispersed into the room

°Needs to be cleaned regularly

°Moist air may be a disadvantage in wet climates

°Cost range is moderate to high

Passive Diffusers

Passive diffusers work with the natural volatility of essential oils. Volatile means that essential oils evaporate easily. Top note oils evaporate more readily. Passive devices are used by placing a few drops of essential oils on an absorbent medium such as a cotton pad or clay object, or by placing a few drops in water on a warming dish over a heat source. Passive diffusers therefore can be further categorized into those using heat and those which do not require heat.

Passive Diffusers Using Heat

Some passive diffusers use heat to accelerate evaporation. Diffusers in this category include oil lamps, electric oil warmers, USB diffusers, and plug in car diffusers. Those units using candles require extra caution due to the presence of an open flame and the flammable nature of essential oils. For this reason never pour essential oils into the warmer *after* the candle has been lit. Candle warmers are also a safety hazard around children and pets, who may knock it over or burn themselves. Electric, USB, or 12V (car) diffusers produce less hazard.

Advantages of Passive Diffusers with Heat

°Many designs available to suit any décor

°Inexpensive

°Thicker oils can be used

°Some are portable (e.g. USB, car)

Disadvantages of Passive Diffusers with Heat

°Properties of essential oils may be altered due to heat

°Components of essential oils may evaporate at different rates

°Burning candles can pose a safety hazard and should not be left unattended

°Non-candle diffusers require a power source

Passive Diffusers without Heat

Passive diffusers that do not use heat work by simple evaporation. They are a natural and inexpensive way to diffuse oils. Examples of passive diffusers include fan diffusers, clay or sandstone diffusers, aromatherapy jewelry, personal inhalers, and room sprays. You can even place a few drops of essential oil on a cotton ball or tissue and let it evaporate.

Advantages of Passive Diffusers without heat:

°No heat is used

°Inexpensive

°Portable

Disadvantages of Passive Diffusers without heat:

°Essential oils may evaporate unevenly, affecting properties

°Weakest scent of all types of diffuser, and scent will fade over the course of the day, especially with top note oils

°Some require special replacement pads (e.g. fan diffusers, some pendants)

°Clay, terracotta or sandstone may require one scent to fade before a new one is applied.

There are many diffusers on the market, and it would be unfair to single out certain products by name in a book. For specific product descriptions and reviews, you can find more information on my website www.diffuseressentials.com.

Questions to ask when choosing a diffuser

Having read through the types of diffusers you may already have a sense of which type of diffuser is right for your needs. If you are still unsure, consider the following factors.

1. **What is your main reason for wanting to diffuse essential oils?**

   °Natural scent-If your primary goal is a fragranced home or car without chemicals, the good news is that any diffuser will work for you. Your decision will be based on how strong a scent you want, the size of the space, and your budget.

   °Enhance mood and emotions-once again any diffuser will work for this purpose, however devices that emit a stronger scent may be more useful than passive diffusers without heat. Your next consideration will be the size of the space and budget.

   °Therapeutic benefits-if you are looking to use aromatherapy as a complementary therapy for a physical or emotional condition, or to prevent disease then a nebulizing diffuser is the best choice. These are also the most expensive models. If your budget doesn't allow for a nebulizing diffuser, consider an ultrasonic diffuser. These units are still efficient at releasing a fine mist of oils into the air at a more moderate price point.

2. **What is the size of the room or space that you will be using the diffuser in?**

   ° Nebulizers and ultrasonics tend to have the best coverage, but output varies from model to model. Most well-known diffusers will list in their specifications the area in square feet that a unit will cover

°If you are moving the unit from room to room, you may want to avoid one with fragile glass parts.

°A passive device will be effective in diffusing oils in a small space such as a car or a bathroom, but would be less suitable for a bedroom or living space

3.   **What level of scent do you desire—a strong, moderate or light aroma?**

°Passive diffusers will create the lightest scent, even though it may be strong initially

°Nebulizing diffusers will create the strongest scent, however these units should only be used for about 10 minutes two to three times a day and in between use, the scent will fade even though the molecules remain suspended in the air for 2-3 hours.

°Ultrasonic diffusers create medium to strong scents depending upon the intensity setting of the machine (often user controlled). Ultrasonic diffusers can be used continuously so if a persistent, even aroma is your goal, this is your best choice.

°Scent level is also dependent on the type of oil used. Some oils will produce a mild scent, while others emit a stronger scent. In Chapter 4 I give the scent strength of my top 10 starter oils.

4.   **Will the unit be used around pets or small children?**

°Around the smallest of children, a nebulizer may be too potent unless used with caution (see Safety chapter discussion of essential oils and children)

°Some oil warmers and nebulizers have glass parts, which may break

°Candle warmers are contraindicated due to an open flame which could cause burns, or be knocked over and start a fire

°Ultrasonics and passive diffusers are the best choice around pets and children

5. What is your budget?

°Diffusers can range from a few dollars to a few hundred dollars

°Low priced options (under $30) include most types of passive diffusers and some ultrasonic models of questionable quality

°Moderately priced options ($30-80) include several ultrasonic models, some fan diffusers, sterling silver aromatherapy jewelry, and a few nebulizing diffusers

°High priced options ($80-400) include nebulizing diffusers and some deluxe ultrasonic diffusers. Many of the higher priced ultrasonic units have special features such as mood lights, or the ability to play music

°Some diffusers have cotton pads which hold the essential oil. These need to be replaced from time to time (though they can be used several times before they need to be tossed out). Although most replacement pads cost a few dollars, some are slightly higher so factor in the ongoing expense of replacement pads.

6. Are you willing to maintain the diffuser?

°Nebulizing diffusers and ultrasonic diffusers require regular cleaning in order to continue functioning properly. Failure to do so can result in the device becoming clogged. This is most important with glass nebulizers. Ultrasonic devices require regular wiping out of the basin that contains the oil and water.

Cleaning diffusers is a simple process so do not be scared off by maintenance, however it must be done regularly. If this is a concern, be sure to look up maintenance instructions for each unit you are considering purchasing. Most manufacturer's post their product's instruction manuals online, and some even have instructional videos online

°Any diffuser with a basin will require at least a wipe out once in a while to prevent a buildup of residue

°Clay or terracotta diffusers may become clogged with oils after a period of time and lose their porosity (and therefore their ability to absorb oils). Most will come with instructions on how to clean the diffuser.

°Diffusers with disposable pads (fan diffusers, car diffusers, some jewelry) require the least maintenance as used pads merely need to be tossed and replaced

Answering these questions should get you well on your way to making an informed decision about whether to purchase an aromatherapy diffuser, and if so, which kind. I hope you now feel confident in choosing a diffuser, selecting some essential oils, and creating your first blends. Aromatherapy is a wonderful way to promote health and well-being and I hope you have found the information in this guide useful.

Bonus: Making your own room spray:

Don't have a diffuser yet? Once you have achieved a blend that you are happy with you can make a room spray. I keep a room spray in my bathroom where the scent of my diffuser does not reach. Making a room spray is easy—you will need:

°A fine mist spritzer bottle (dark glass is best)

°A neutral spirit such as high proof vodka or pure grain alcohol

°Distilled water

°Your essential oil blend

For every ounce of finished product the proportions are 12 drops of essential oil, 1 tsp. alcohol and 1 ounce of distilled water. Combine the essential oils and alcohol first. Essential oils are not water soluble, but they are partially soluble in alcohol. After blending the oils and alcohol, add your distilled water. I recommend giving the mixture a quick shake before each use to ensure that the essential oils are evenly distributed.

Thank you for choosing this book. If you found this book useful, please do me the favor of taking a moment to leave a review at Amazon. Your feedback is essential, no pun intended, for independent authors.

You can find more information about diffusing essential oils at my website www.diffuseressentials.com and I invite you to ask questions or leave comments there about anything you didn't understand or want more information about.

If you have any suggestions for future editions of this book, please contact me through my website http://www.diffuseressentials.com/aboutlegal/contact/

If you participate in social media, telling the world about this book is the greatest compliment you can give and I would sincerely appreciate it.

To your health,

Joy

Glossary

Analgesic: relieves pain

Anesthetic: blocks pain sensations

Anti-Aging: prevents or diminishes signs of aging

Antibacterial: fights against bacteria

Anticatarrhal: prevents or alleviates buildup and discharge of mucus in mucus membranes such as nose and throat

Anticlotting: inhibits blood clotting

Antiemetic: inhibits vomiting

Antifungal: fights against fungus

Antihistaminic: inhibits the production or action of histamines

Anti-Inflammatory: reduces inflammation

Antimicrobial: reduces microbes

Antineuralgic: relieving neuralgic pain (which is a sharp nerve pain)

Antioxidant: inhibits oxidation (oxidation leads to free radicals)

Antiparasitic: fights against parasites

Antiputrefactive: preserves against decay

Antirheumatic: relieves rheumatism (which causes stiff muscles and swollen joints)

Antiseptic: kills microbes

Antispasmodic: relieves muscle spasms

Antiviral: fights against viruses

Apertif: stimulates the appetite

Aphrodisiac: stimulates sexual desire

Aromatic: emits a pleasant smell

Astringent: tightens the skin

Bactericidal: kills bacteria

Carminative: relieves flatulence

Cell Proliferant: encourages multiplication of cells

Cephalic-relates to the head

Cholagogue: stimulates flow of bile

Cicatrizant: promotes wound healing

Decongestant: eases nasal congestion

Deodorant: conceals or takes away body odors

Depurative: purifying or detoxifying

Diaphoretic: causes perspiration

Digestive: aids in digestion

Diuretic: causes increase in urine output

Emmenagogue: stimulates menstrual flow

Expectorant: promotes expelling of mucus

Febrifuge: reduces fever

Fungicidal: kills funus

Galactagogue: promotes flow of milk

Insect Repellant: repels insects

Insecticide: kills insects

Laxative: stimulates purging of the bowels

Nervine: calms nerves

Regenerative: restores and renews

Regulatory: puts in order

Rubefacient: causes skin redness, increase in circulation to skin

Sedative: calms or promotes sleep

Stimulant: arouses or quickens functions

Stomachic: promoting appetite and helping digestion

Styptic: stops bleeding

Sudorific: causes perspiration

Tonic: promotes a feeling of well being

Uterine: affects the uterus

Vermifuge: anti-parastitic

Vulnerary: helps heal wounds

Works Cited

1. Watt, Martin. Essential Oils: Their lack of skin absorption, but effectiveness via inhalation. http://www.naturehelps.com/agora/skinabso.htm

2. Doran, Morden, Dunn, Edwards-Jones, 2009. Vapour-phase activities of essential oils against antibiotic sensitive and resistant bacteria including MRSA. http://www.ncbi.nlm.nih.gov/pubmed/19292822

3. BBC News. Essential oils 'combat superbug.' http://news.bbc.co.uk/2/hi/uk_news/england/manchester/6471475.s tm

4. National Association for Holistic Aromatherapy. http://www.naha.org/explore-aromatherapy/safety/

5. Learning about EO's (website). Essential oils and children. http://www.learningabouteos.com/index.php/2014/02/07/essentialoils-and-children/

6. Jones, Beth (2014). 600 Aromatherapy Recipes for Beauty, Health & Home.

7. Web M.D. (website). Lavender. http://www.webmd.com/vitaminssupplements/ingredientmono-838lavender.aspx?activeingredientid=838&activeingredientname=lave nder

8. Lewith, Godfrey, Prescott (2005). A single-blinded, randomized pilot study evaluating the aroma of Lavandula augustifolia [sic] as a treatment for mild insomnia.
http://www.ncbi.nlm.nih.gov/pubmed/16131287

9. Lee & Lee (2006). Effects of lavender aromatherapy on insomnia and depression in women college students.
http://www.ncbi.nlm.nih.gov/pubmed/16520572

10. Buchbauer, Jirovetz, Jager, Dietrich, Plank (1991). Aromatherapy: evidence for sedative effects of the essential oil of lavender after inhalation. http://www.ncbi.nlm.nih.gov/pubmed/1817516

11. Sayorwan, Siripornpanich, Piriyapunyaporn, Hongratanaworakit, Kotchabhakdi, Ruangrungsi (2012). The effects of lavender oil inhalation on emotional states, autonomic nervous system, and brain electrical activity.
http://www.ncbi.nlm.nih.gov/pubmed/22612017

12. Sasannejad, Saeedi, Shoeibi, Gorji, Abbasi, Foroughipour (2012). Lavender essential oil in the treatment of migraine headache: A placebo-controlled clinical trial.
http://www.karger.com/Article/Abstract/335249

13. Self (Website). Lemon peel, raw nutrition facts & calories.
http://nutritiondata.self.com/facts/fruits-and-fruit-juices/1941/2

14. Kiecolt-Glaser, Graham, Malarkey, Porter, Lemeshow, Glaser (2008). Olfactory influences on mood and autonomic, endocrine, and immune function.
http://www.ncbi.nlm.nih.gov/pubmed/18178322

15. E-how (website). What does norepinephrine do?
http://www.ehow.com/about_5548212_norepinephrine-do.html

16. Bigos, Wasiela, Kalemba, Sienkiewicz (2012). Antimicrobial activity of geranium oil against clinical strains of Staphylococcus aureus. http://www.ncbi.nlm.nih.gov/pubmed/22929626

17. Tate (1997). Peppermint oil: a treatment for postoperative nausea.
http://www.ncbi.nlm.nih.gov/pubmed/9378876

18. Jung & Lee (2004). Effects of aroma oil inhalation on nausea, vomiting and anorexia in cancer patients receiving chemotherapy.
http://www.koreamed.org/SearchBasic.php?RID=0094JKAAN%2
F 2004.16.1.135&DT=1

19. WebMD (Website). Peppermint.
http://www.webmd.com/vitaminssupplements/ingredientmono-705peppermint.aspx?activeingredientid=705&activeingredientnam
e=p eppermint

20. Moss, Hewitt, Moss, Wesnes (2006). Modulation of cognitive performance and mood by aromas of peppermint and ylang-ylang.
http://www.greenmedinfo.com/article/aroma-peppermint-enhancesmemory-and-increases-alertness-human-subjects

21. Sadlon & Lamson (2010). Immune-modifying and antimicrobial effects of Eucalyptus oil and simple inhalation devices.

http://www.ncbi.nlm.nih.gov/pubmed/20359267

22. Gobel, Schmidt, Soyka (1994). Effect of peppermint and eucalyptus oil preparations on neurophysiological and experimental algesimetric headache parameters.
http://www.ncbi.nlm.nih.gov/pubmed/7954745

23. Fu, Zu, Chen, Shi, Wang, Sun, Efferth (2007). Antimicrobial activity of clove and rosemary essential oils alone and in combination.
http://onlinelibrary.wiley.com/doi/10.1002/ptr.2179/abstract

24. Moss, Cook, Wesnes, Duckett (2003). Aromas of Rosemary and Lavender essential oils differentially affect cognition and mood in healthy adults.
http://informahealthcare.com/doi/abs/10.1080/0020745039016190 3

25. McCaffrey, Thomas, Kinzelman (2009). The effects of Lavender and Rosemary essential oils on test taking anxiety among graduate nursing students.
http://journals.lww.com/hnpjournal/Abstract/2009/03000/The_Effe cts_of_Lavender_and_Rosemary_Essential.5.aspx

26. Mateusz, Oleg, Majewski, Skwarlo-Sonta (2005). Tea tree oil inhalations modify immunity in mice.
http://www.researchgate.net/publication/26596336_Tea_tree_oil_in halations_modify_immunity_in_mice

27. Carson, Hammer, Riley (2006). Melaleuca alternifolia (Tea Tree) oil: A review of antimicrobial and other medicinal properties.
http://www.ncbi.nlm.nih.gov/pmc/articles/PMC1360273/

28. Prabuseenivasan, Jayakumar, Ignacimuthu (2006). In vitro antibacterial activity of some plant essential oils. http://www.biomedcentral.com/1472-6882/6/39

29. British Psychological Society (2013). Rosemary aroma may help you to remember to do things. http://www.sciencedaily.com/releases/2013/04/130409091104.htm

37916186R00049

Made in the USA
Middletown, DE
12 December 2016